THRIVING
IN THE NHS

THRIVING IN THE NHS

AN INTERNATIONAL MEDICAL GRADUATE'S GUIDE TO STARTING OUT IN THE NHS

IBIFUNKE PEGBA-OTEMOLU

THRIVING IN THE NHS
An International Medical Graduate's Guide
To Starting Out In The Nhs

Copyright © 2020
Ibifunke Pegba-Otemolu

Cover Illustration: Olajumoke Adegunle
Editor: Olakitan Jokodola

Published by Afterplab, a subsidiary of
Eldorado Medic Jobs Limited

To my wonderful God, who blesses me in immeasurable ways.

To my husband, who believed enough in my aspirations to try long distance marriage.

To my lovely children who have become 'my why'.

To my amazing family and friends like family, you lift me up.

EDITORS

Dr Ifechi Ezumba
BSc. Human Biology, MbChB, MPH, GP Trainee

'Sola Fatoke MBA
Senior Clinical Fellow, Essex Cardiothoracic Centre

Dr Gbemisola Oyeneyin
MBBS, Obstetrics and Gynaecology Trainee

CONTENTS

FOREWORD

I met Dr Ibifunke Pegba-Otemolu as a junior doctor as she rotated through the surgical department where I work as a consultant surgeon and governor for the Oxford University Hospitals Foundation. She was always enthusiastic, well read and remarkably calm whilst she perfectly balanced a busy home life and full-time surgical career. Toward the end of her time in Oxford we served on the Board of Governors for the Trust.

Having worked in the National Health Service for over 20 years there is little doubt about the reliance of the NHS on foreign health professionals to keep it running – the last 30 years has seen a boom of doctors from all over the world coming across to help keep up with the demands of our NHS. This book hits on key themes of the difficulties faced from the minute one embarks upon a career in the NHS and the struggles and tribulations one can expect to encounter.

I recall junior doctors telling me about lengthy battles with GMC red tape and immigration hoops that need to be jumped through which provide financial and time-consuming obstacles. Once in the UK structure one then needs to negotiate the turbulent training system with its own demands and difficulties. Courses come at a premium for those not recognised as 'UK trainees' and cost of living can be higher than expected in some areas of the UK.

This book gives a breakdown of what life can be like in the first few years and acts as an excellent survival guide for any doctor coming into the UK system. It systematically goes through the journey to get to the NHS system, it traverses the minefield that can be the job and breaks these down into bitesize paragraphs, giving concise information. Whilst there is nothing like real life experience, I feel this book gives the reader an idea of NHS life along with hints and tricks on survival.

Up to date guidance is given on key topics such as bullying where new roles such as 'Freedom to Speak Up Guardian' are talked about – so that you know who to turn to when feeling bullied. These are drawn from personal experiences from Dr Pegba-Otemolu who has lived and thrived in the UK system becoming an invaluable and dependable doctor in the department who rose to the rank of governor with her keen interest in hospital management.

The journey through the NHS is difficult for UK trainees – let alone for those who come from abroad. Sadly, a profound deep-rooted culture exists within the NHS and 'outsiders' are still treated differently. Whilst this is slowly changing over time – we are still many years away from being where we should be. In the meanwhile, guides like this book help doctors – UK trained and abroad to settle into the job and know where and how to get help.

It is a highly recommended read for all those starting life in the NHS at any level and from any background. Interestingly, at a personal level, I feel it is valuable read for anyone working in the NHS as it gives generic information for all but certain chapters also give some insight into what some doctors have to go through to join the NHS. With more understanding and empathy, the NHS can be a better work environment for all.

Shad Khan

PREFACE

I moved to the United Kingdom in the winter of 2016, pregnant and armed with ambitions to be a plastic surgery trainee and subsequently, embark on a fellowship in breast surgery in the United States. I had read a few blog posts about specialty applications in plastic surgery and thought I had all the information I needed to apply the following year. I was wrong!

I was fortunate to find senior colleagues who took me 'under their wings' and in some cases, I found mentors to guide me. The time I spent with these people was invaluable in the planning of my professional life.

As an international medical graduate, you need to learn things that locally trained graduates in the UK take for granted. For instance, recruitment is centralised and annual for many specialties; it is more advantageous to get into training at core specialty level than at specialty level. Moreover, you can be overqualified to get into a training programme.

Now that you have decided to pursue a medical career as an International Medical Graduate (IMG) in the UK, what next?

Are you familiar with the career path? Do you know the required procedure to experience growth on your journey?

In this book, I will share the knowledge I have gained by way of experience and guidance from seniors. I hope it provides light that smoothens your passage.

CHAPTER 1

WHY ARE YOU MOVING?

People decide to move for various reasons. It is important to define your reasons because it will guide your decision making for the type of jobs you apply to, whether or not you apply for training programmes, how you select the training programmes if you decide to go into training and even determine the type of accommodation you get.

My decision to move was guided by the desire to gain surgical skills and get into a training programme. It dictated the kinds of jobs I applied for, the decision to change jobs and the requirements I looked out for while applying for jobs.

If you are moving with the hope of getting into training, there are a few things to note before starting your job application process. First, consider your level of experience. There are various levels at which an International Medical Graduate (IMG) can access the

UK system – as a Foundation year 1 or 2 trainee, a senior house officer (SHO) or as a specialty doctor (senior registrar level). The application processes for all differ and will be discussed in detail in subsequent chapters.

However, in this chapter, it is important to understand your options, based on your level of experience, in order to streamline your focus during job application. Basically, the application processes for different jobs are not the same. So, it is important to know what you intend to achieve and understand your options, in order to maintain focus during your job search, rather than applying for jobs randomly.

If you completed medical school and have less than one year experience, you may consider applying for eligibility for Foundation training through the UK Foundation Programme (UKFP) office. If you have completed one year training post medical school, you may be eligible for F2 jobs. Your eligibility is assessed by the UKFP office.

Housemanship, house job and Foundation training are synonymous. In the UK it is a two-year training programme and the selection process is centralised. As a non-UK and non-EEA (European Economic Area) trained medical graduate, your eligibility for the Foundation programme is confirmed through the UK Foundation Programme (UKFP) Office. This process typically begins the year before starting your Foundation training. The processes and requirements are regularly reviewed; so, stay updated.

When an application is sent to the UKFP, a decision about the candidate's eligibility to apply for Foundation training is made by the office. Note that there is a window of opportunity to appeal the decision of the UKFP before the application for Foundation opens. Candidates may either apply for Foundation programmes alone or alongside Academic Foundation programmes. A link to the guidance for UKFP eligibility programme can be found in the additional resources section of this book. Therefore, begin preparation ahead of the release of eligibility criteria, using the previous year's resources, to afford yourself adequate time to collate your information.

The eligibility for Foundation training application is one out of three requirements. The other two are a provisional license to practice, which is obtainable from the GMC (General Medical Council) and proof of proficiency in English language. Applicants are required to have passed the Professional and Linguistic Assessments Board

(PLAB) examination, in order to obtain a provisional license from the GMC.

All applications are made through Oriel, which is a web-based platform used in the UK to apply for training posts. Sign up on Oriel and enable notifications for applications you will be interested in. If you have completed your Foundation training and already granted full licence to practice, you can apply for either Senior House Officer (SHO) or registrar roles. However, if you have less than three years post graduate medical experience, it is advisable to stick to SHO roles.

With more than three years' experience, you may decide either to apply for more senior roles or not. It is important to state here that the expectations for knowledge are very high in the UK and in most specialties, the UK is more advanced than the country an IMG has trained in.

For that reason, it is useful to spend at least six months in an SHO role to get familiar with the system. In most specialties, the consultants will be pleased to get you into a more senior role once they can vouch for your expertise. For very senior clinicians, it is probably safe to go straight into a specialty doctor role as you will have juniors covering tasks that you have lost familiarity with.

After deciding your preferred job level, choose the specialty areas you are comfortable working in. If you aspire for specialty training, then, visit the Oriel website which has the recruitment requirements for each of the specialties. Review the requirements for the specialty of your choice. It has details of the maximum amount of time (excluding Foundation training) that you should spend in a specialty in order to be eligible to apply. This amount of time includes overseas experience. Therefore, if taking a job in that specialty will put you over the limit, apply in a different specialty.

Applying for a job in a specialty different from your aspiration may make it difficult to achieve the requirements laid out in the person specification for that specialty. The important thing is balance. You can look for roles that have cross-cover commitments. This means that during your on- call shifts, you cover multiple specialties.

For example, my first role was as an orthopaedic SHO. My cross-cover commitments included urology, general surgery and gynaecology. I showed my commitment to general surgery during my call duties. Through the relationship I developed with consultants in general surgery, I got the opportunity to be involved in a multi-centre audit, a case study and an international audit. All these helped me to build my portfolio for general surgery

Another option is to take on jobs that have rotations. For example, a two-year contract with a Trust that gives a year each in two different specialties. If you take on a contract with the intention of rotating, ensure it is clearly stated that you will rotate and the rotation dates are given. Trusts have been known to deny doctors the opportunity to rotate due to shortages.

I had taken on my first job based on the agreement that I would rotate to general surgery in the second year. When the time was approaching, I was told that the team could not accommodate me. This led to seeking a job in general surgery in a different Trust.

Another job type that enables you avoid racking up time in your specialty of choice is teaching fellowships. They are usually offered by specialties in Teaching Hospitals.

CHOOSING A SPONSOR

This section is for IMGs who are the principal applicant in the family. IMGs on spousal visas do not require sponsors. A sponsor provides a certificate of sponsorship (CoS) which is a unique number that can be used to apply for a Tier 2 visa. For clinical jobs, there are two main options for visa sponsorship – an NHS Trust and a locum agency.

For private hospitals, the locum agency sponsors the visa. In the case of NHS, the NHS organisation is the visa sponsor but the candidate is shortlisted by the locum agency.

NHS jobs and the levels at which most people can apply have been previously described. For private organisations, doctors are called Resident Medical Officers. They offer work commitments in weekly blocks - one week on and another week off or two weeks as the case may be. They are also offered in different specialties. The services are typically provided in private hospitals around the UK.

The pay generally tends to be less than the NHS roles but the time off affords flexibility to either make additional income or study for examination. It can be beneficial to apply for jobs on the NHS website alongside applications through the agencies. The agencies may contact you through programmes organised in your home country, via professional sites like LinkedIn or they can also be found through search engines.

If you secure a job through an agency, a recruitment officer will be assigned to you to provide guidance and support all through the application process.

NHS jobs are aggregated on the NHS job website. On the website, filters can be applied to the search. The filters can help with selecting the seniority level of the jobs that you want to apply to, geographic location, salary and specialty. To complete the application, there will be initial pages which obtain background information like demographics, visa status and previous jobs.

For the referee section, ensure you have obtained permission from the referees and the contact information provided, particularly the email address, is in regular use by the referees. Delays from referees can slow down your employment process.

The supporting evidence section is the most important part of the application and determines whether your application will be shortlisted or not. It is advisable to modify this section for every application. To optimise this section, carefully examine the job description and the person specification. Then, respond to the questions in a manner that showcases your skills and expertise in meeting their expectations. For example, if applying to a job where you will oversee the wards, showcase your experience(s) of leading ward rounds in previous jobs.

IMGs may struggle with questions such as demonstrating a time they managed a change in the past. The temptation is to believe you have no experience that can be used. Invariably, everyone would have had an opportunity to improve the way something is done. No matter how small that change was, it is still an achievement. Think carefully about it and you will find a good example.

For my first application, I used my experience from a small renal dialysis unit where I had worked. I had introduced interdepartmental meetings which improved communication between staff.

The other area that can create anxiety is questions about quality improvement and audit experience. If you have no experience, it is safe to be honest and state that you aspire to gain this experience if given the opportunity to join the organisation.

In the free text section where you are asked for any additional information, sell yourself. Give a brief summary of your work experience and education, and how they prepared you to be the most suitable candidate for the role. Then, outline the opportunities you look forward to, if you join the organisation. In addition, explain why you think you are the best fit for the role. Once you have completed an application, save it as a template so that the effort is reduced for subsequent applications. Avoid the temptation to use the same application for all the positions you apply to. Rather, modify the supporting information so that it suits the person specification for each role you apply for.

INTERVIEWS, OFFERS AND REJECTION

Once you are shortlisted, prepare adequately for the interview. The interviewers will ask clinical questions around the role you are being interviewed for. Therefore, be ready to demonstrate your clinical knowledge, particularly managing of emergencies.

For example, I applied to an endocrine surgery job and was asked how I would manage hypocalcaemia after a thyroidectomy. There may also be questions about dealing with difficult situations like having to make a complaint about a colleague, cancel a clinic, why you want the job, your strengths, weaknesses, etc.

Any standard interview preparation will serve. The important thing is to prepare answers, practice and be in the right frame of mind.

If you get the long rejection email that ends in "unfortunately you were not selected", it hurts; but, it is not the end. Write an appreciation letter and ask for feedback. Then, use the feedback to prepare better for your next application.

When you receive a congratulatory message, before you accept and the organisation issues a CoS, ensure you have been made a fair offer in terms of your salary, leave and reimbursement for relocation. You will be interacting with the staff services office during the process of being shortlisted and recruited; so ask all necessary questions. While the staff services team do not set out to be dishonest, they may not be fully open in terms of all the benefits that are available to you. So, ensure you are knowledgeable about the right questions to ask, especially the financial aspects.

Consider the following:

- Is the salary scale you are being offered commensurate with your years of experience? During the application process, you should have researched the salary scale commensurate with your level of experience. Check to ascertain that the salary being offered is right for you. Be aware that if you are offered a salary grade lower than your years of experience, you can negotiate.
- Is reimbursement of relocation cost available?

Reimbursement of relocation cost is usually available if you are moving from a different country. Depending on your level and where you are moving to within the country, it may also be available. Ask! If what you are offered is significantly lower than the projected expenses, then, negotiate for more. If some money is due to you, process the payment and make sure it is paid. Follow-up is essential.

Sometimes, the process can be more stressful than expected but it will be satisfying when the payment is made.

- Is it compulsory to resume on the start date stipulated? Choosing a start date can be daunting. As an IMG, especially if you are relocating to take up your first job, you are required to choose a start date. This date is used on the certificate of sponsorship (CoS) issued by your employer.

The start date on your CoS is not binding. After you have obtained your visa, your staff services contact will ask about your start date. This helps them plan the rota. Before you choose a date, consider your personal circum-stances well. Do not feel under pressure to pick a close date. Pick a date that realistically allows you fulfil all your obligations and arrive in good health of mind and body to resume your new job.

In choosing your start date, also ask when the Trust has inductions. It is in your best interest to complete your induction before you start working, especially if it is your first NHS job. If the Trust you are joining have staff shortages, they may advise you to start working without induction. I strongly discourage this!

CHAPTER 2

THE MOVE

The visa issued in your passport is called a vignette and it allows you into the country to pick up your Biometric Residence Permit. The employer will need to view your passport and Biometric Residence Permit, in order to make copies before you are allowed to start work. When planning for your travel, check the weather report. This will guide your preparation, in terms of getting appropriate clothes for the weather.

ACCOMMODATION

Most hospitals have accommodation facilities. If you are travelling with your family, inform the staff services team, as family accommodation is sometimes available. When it is not, you may be required to make arrangements for your accommodation. In some Trusts, even though it is not hospital accommodation, support may be available for temporary accommodation for your family - financial support to pay for the accommodation and contacts of temporary accommodation options near the hospital.

For contingency purposes, plan for the cost of an extra week at the temporary accommodation, in case things take longer than expected.

Finding the right accommodation can be tricky, especially when moving with your family. In view of this, there are a number of factors to consider. For instance, consider how much you value privacy, cleanliness (if you have to share living areas) and things you are willing to trade off such as cost of transportation versus living on the premises. If you are alone, shared hospital accommodation can provide a cheaper option if you do not mind sharing living spaces.

Hospital accommodation may be cheaper and more convenient, if you do not plan to move immediately. It may also afford you the opportunity to acclimatise to the area/environment before you choose where to settle. If proximity to work is not an important consideration, then, offsite accommodation is an option. Websites like Rightmove and Zoopla are good places to start your search.

For example, the hospital accommodation in the first place I lived was a 3-bedroom old creaky house. All bills included, it cost about 1065 GBP. I moved during winter and I was pregnant. I did not have the energy to search for offsite accommodation using public transportation in the cold weather. So, I opted for hospital accommodation.

Also, I was not interested in shared accommodation, even though it was cheaper. This was because I wanted the freedom of having my own space. The hospital should have reimbursed me for the accommodation in the first month but they never did and I wasn't aware I could ask. Do not make the same mistake!

After my maternity leave, I found a spacious, modern, furnished two-bedroom flat. The total cost of rent and bills was about 900 GBP. An added bonus was its proximity to the city centre. However, the downside was that I had to pay for transportation to work. Notwithstanding, it was an improvement comfort wise.

When choosing your accommodation, you may wonder at the difference in cost between furnished and unfurnished property. Furnished options seem more expensive than unfurnished property. The cost savings from getting an unfurnished place is usually spent on furnishing the property. The cost of moving acquired property, if moving becomes necessary, should also be taken into consideration when weighing options.

Furniture can be obtained with full price paid upfront or in monthly instalments from stores like Ikea or far cheaper from charity stores, Facebook or other media market places. Not all items sold cheaper are used; you may find new furniture. Be sure to verify sellers and meet safely to exchange goods and money. The steps involved in securing a rental place include the process of reference checks. Usually, your staff services contact will act as your referee to the landlord or agents.

Consider hiring a cleaner before you move in. Most places are nice and clean when you move in while some just look clean. Hiring a cleaner means, you can unpack straight away without having to clean grease out of cupboards or worry about unclogging drainages. The balance here is cost versus convenience.

During your time in the property, promptly report any fault that develops. If you have a good landlord and agent, it will get fixed quickly at no cost to you. Treat the property like it is yours. This has two benefits. First, it gets you into the habit of being careful, which will serve you when you buy your property. Secondly, it reduces the likelihood of losing a significant part of your deposit when you move out.

Bills are usually inclusive with your rent for hospital accommodation. On the other hand, off site accommodation will not be the same. When searching for options, ask locals like colleagues or your contact in staff services about safe areas. If you have children of school age, ask about areas with good schools. Also, research online as a lot of comparison websites exist to guide people. Mumsnet is a useful resource.

Council tax is tax that is paid to your local council monthly. The amount paid is guided by the tax band the property you are renting belongs to. Some factors that influence the cost include the size of the property, its location and whether it is occupied by a single adult. It is helpful to know the council tax band of the property before you rent it, as this will influence how much you will be spending in addition to rent.

If you are the only adult living in the property, you can obtain a single person discount by applying to the council. The council website will publish the days waste disposal is carried out in your neighbourhood.

Other bills include energy, electricity, gas, internet and water. For internet access, check online to find out the providers with the best speed for the area where you will be living. You will learn that services are not always available as soon as you need them; so, early planning helps. This is particularly important for internet access. As soon as you have an agreement with the landlord or agents, even while waiting for final checks and handover of the keys, order your internet. That way, it will arrive in the quickest possible time.

There are also options for same day service depending on the provider. The important thing is to sort it early, so you can get your internet access as soon as possible.

When you are moving out, I strongly advise you use the cleaning agents recommended by your landlord. Chances are the price will seem steep and you could get a cheaper option, which may be yourself or a cheaper cleaner. However, any dissatisfaction with the service rendered means additional costs to you.

It is easier to pay the service charge of the recommended cleaner, because you will not be expected to pay if the job is not satisfactorily done. What if things go wrong? When you move in, you will be given a lot of documents. One of them is a

Tenancy Deposit Scheme pamphlet or pdf document. It gives you guidelines on what to do if your landlord attempts to withhold your deposit unfairly. Due to the possibility of this occurring, be sure to document all communication between you and agents.

Typically, it will be via emails; so, do not delete them. In the event that your communication is via a phone call, follow it up with an email detailing your discussion. Do not give in to bullying tactics which are sometimes employed. Make it clear that you are aware of your rights.

STARTING AT WORK

Before you start work that interfaces with patients, occupational health will conduct blood tests for infectious diseases. This can take a few days. It is useful to spend these days setting up a bank account, applying for National Insurance (NI) number and registering with your local General Practitioner.

Your interviewers would have formed opinions about you and shared them with your new colleagues ahead of your arrival. Now, you would not know whether the information casts you in a positive or negative light and there is no point speculating. Do your best to create good first impressions when you meet the team.

If you get formally introduced, that is wonderful and a sign that you have probably chosen a good place. If you are not introduced to team mates, introduce yourself. Let everyone know that it is your first week and your first job in the NHS. This way, people are more eager to offer help when they see you struggling.

For first timers, some Trusts will offer you the opportunity to shadow a colleague for some time. It may seem odd to you especially if you are very experienced. However, it gives both you and your employers time to adjust before you see patients. Use the time judiciously as you can learn a lot. The length of time varies by Trust and speciality. If you are a senior and not given this opportunity, request to shadow a colleague on call before you take that responsibility.

Being on call often involves an increased scope of work such as receiving referrals and attending to ward based referrals. It is important to understand what the on call commitments are before you start taking on call shifts.

SOCIALISING

Social rules and how you gain friends are different around the world, even though general principles tend to be the same. Here are few don'ts that can help you blend in quicker:

- Do not go to lunch alone. Rather, have lunch dates with your colleagues. You will get to know them quicker and also learn important things that you will need to get by.
- Do not make a cup of tea or drink water without offering others as well.
- Do not always be the person who accepts free coffee but never offers to buy for others.
- Do not be missing from team events every time.

Try as you might, there will be people you cannot seem to please. That is ok! You cannot be everyone's cup of tea. Learn to be fine with that. In some cases, it may be due to the colour of your skin; although that is not ok, learn to pick your battles.

Depending on the part of the UK you reside, the friendliness of locals and their willingness to accept diverse skin tones may vary. For example, from my personal experience, Grimsby in the north of England has very friendly locals who treat ethnic minority professionals with kindness and respect. In Weston-Super-Mare, South West of England, the locals are not really welcoming to foreigners. It can be a difficult transition to suddenly become a label other than how you have always identified yourself and to realise that you are not simply a person to others.

You now come with a label. Do not take it personal. You are not the first to go through this struggle and are unlikely to be the last. Take it in your stride. Call out people when things go over the top and ignore subtle aggressors. If you respond every single time, you lose your joy and become identified unfairly as the one who always throws the race card.

DRIVING

When relocating, take along a valid driver's license. You are permitted to drive with it for the first twelve months after you become a resident. Subsequently, you will be required to get a provisional driver's license, which is also needed for driving lessons.

The driving test is in two parts – the theory which comprises of questions and hazard perception testing, and the practical test. Be sure to practice for the hazard perception test as well when preparing. The theory examination is valid for two years within which you are expected to pass the practical.

During the practical, you will drive around with the test administrator. You will decide if you wish to be accompanied by your instructor or not for the test. It is helpful to start by taking the theory examination.

This helps you to get familiar with the rules of driving in the UK and the meaning of the road signs. Once this is cleared, you can start your driving lessons. Always have a test date that is convenient for you and your instructor, and be realistic.

Though it can be tempting to choose an instructor from online resources, I strongly advise you use an instructor that can be vouched for by a colleague. Instructors may have hidden motives; an instructor may fail to teach you aspects you need to know for the test such as how to come to an emergency stop. Also, he may keep taking you for more hours of driving while telling you about not being ready for the test, even when you feel otherwise.

It is important to add that instructors are not permitted to go beyond a maximum number of student failures; otherwise, they will be investigated. So, it is in their best interest that you pass. Lastly, do not hesitate to change your instructor if you have doubts.

FINANCES

It is important to plan to have funds available in your first month. This is because funds available to you from your Trust may take some time to process. Keep receipts related to your cost of relocation such as airline fares, travel to Trust, and accommodation. You will need them to claim refunds.

Opening a bank account as soon as possible is helpful. Some banks have online account opening facilities while others give appointments. Do some research and contact the bank early so you can set up an account. The staff services team will need your bank details, so it can be forwarded to the payroll department.

In order to work and be paid in the UK, a National Insurance (NI) number is required. This can be obtained by applying for it. Instructions for the application can be found on gov.uk website. Once you have this number, it should be given to the staff services team.

Taxation takes a significant proportion of your earnings. The income tax deducted is based on your tax code. When you receive your payslip, check the tax code and confirm it is appropriate. Information about the tax codes can also be found on gov.uk website. The income tax is likely to increase in the initial months until it reaches the maximum for your income level and plateaus.

Always check your payslip and clarify doubts with the payroll department. If the wrong tax code is applied and you pay more than necessary, it is possible to request a refund.

Credit cards are not the devil and should not be avoided. They help you build your credit history, which will come in handy in future when you want to make purchases using credit facilities. Having a good credit history will improve your eligibility. It is wise not to rack up credit card bills as the interest rate can be quite high. Look out for notifications from your bank to increase your credit limit automatically. Decide cautiously whether or not to take this opportunity.

Another important factor that helps with credit ratings is being on the electoral register or simply put, registering to vote.

Developing a savings culture is important, as expenses pile up quickly. These expenses may include visa fees, courses, examination, driving lessons, mortgages, cars, childcare, relocation (if you have to move) and deposits for accommodation. Most people I know dealt with financial needs as they came up; however, there are financial advisers who specifically cater to the needs of medics. It might be worth speaking to one, in order to have a more robust plan in place.

VISA

Most IMGs start out on Tier 2 visas that are granted for a fixed duration. It is important to pay attention to the date the visa expires, as it will guide actions that need to be taken. If you intend to apply for training, preparation will consume time and energy; and it is unlikely you can apply for a new job at the same time. Ensure you have a good relationship with your current employer so that if your application for training is unsuccessful, there is the opportunity to remain in your current job.

If your training application is successful, you will be required to apply for a visa. It may be necessary to demonstrate that you have the maintenance funds saved for this visa application. Be aware of the visa requirements when applying for the post. If your family need visas as well, it may be possible to apply for theirs at a later date. This can help spread the expenses over time. Remember to read the rules for the most up to date information. For IMGs, the key to success is preparation.

If you intend to stay on the same job and your visa is due to expire, confirmation of your contract renewal should be received from your clinical lead. Visa renewal of less than one year duration is not financially reasonable, because it may lead to paying for visa again within a short time. The human resource team should be able to issue documentation for your application once you are within three months of the expiry of the visa.

Applying early means that you can avoid paying the high cost for urgent applications (same day decisions or within 30 days).

If you would like to change jobs, start searching at least nine months before your visa expires or before the date you would like to start a new job. It takes time to secure a new job considering the application process, short listing, interviews, agreements in terms of salaries, visa applications, moving and settling.

As at the time of writing this book, medical jobs were on the shortage occupation list. This took off the requirement to fulfil a Resident Labour Market Test (RLMT). That requirement meant that employers had to advertise a job for 28 days and prove their inability to find a British or EEA candidate as qualified or better qualified to fill up the role. This change partially levelled the playing field; yet, made jobs more competitive. The rules change regularly, so check before you make plans.

After 5 years in the UK on a Tier 2 visa, you cannot re-apply for the same visa. At this point, you are eligible to apply for permanent residency called

Indefinite Leave to Remain (ILR). At present, you should not have been out of the country for longer than 180 days in any year in the preceding five years. A year in this case begins from the date you first arrived the country on a Tier 2 visa. The ILR application is expensive, so it is useful to start saving for it many years in advance.

Twelve months after the ILR is obtained, eligibility opens to apply to be a British citizen. Although these are the current immigration rules, they are in a state of flux. Stay up to date!

CHAPTER 3

ON THE JOB

This chapter addresses getting to know the actual workings of the system. We will examine challenges with IT, new technologies, cultural differences, dealing with bullies, changing jobs and other helpful tips.

Prior to the Corona virus pandemic, the NHS had a fairly strict bare below the elbows policy. This meant that staff were not expected to wear clothes which extended below their elbows or accessories like watches. Ties were also frowned upon. Rings, if they were worn, were to be plain bands.

During the pandemic, staff were expected to wear scrubs at work and not plain clothes. It is useful to find out what the acceptable attire is before you resume work. Most Trusts will provide scrubs or uniforms where they expect staff to dress as such. If the scrubs or uniforms are dispensed from vending machines, ask for access codes or other required information needed to obtain the attire.

DEALING WITH TECHNOLOGY

Different people have varied levels of experience using electronic records. In most UK hospitals, there is some degree of use of electronic medical records but the extent tends to vary. Most hospitals have electronic laboratory services. It is very important to learn its use and this should be prioritised. You will need access to the systems and training on how to use them; pay attention to the training especially the shortcuts. The time saved can improve your efficiency.

Understand the way laboratory requests are made in your facility. Sometimes, all requests are electronic while some Trusts combine handwritten and electronic requests. Understanding how specimen gets to the laboratory is important, particularly for specimen that needs urgent processing.

Pod systems are pneumatic driven delivery systems that transport plastic tubes within the hospital. They are employed in many Trusts for delivering specimen and there are usually peculiarities when using them. For example, highly infectious specimen cannot be sent through them and they may not be reliable in an emergency. Learn about the systems that obtain in your facility as soon as you start.

Another piece of technology you may struggle with is the blood gas machine. The level of interaction with this machine is dependent on seniority. Senior clinicians request the blood gas test while more junior clinicians do the legwork that gets the test done. The blood gas machines are a scarce resource with several units needing to share them.

Two things are required – knowledge of the location of the machines and access to them. Access to the machines is usually by a login or barcode which is granted after completing the training. If you are starting as a junior doctor, ensure you have this sorted before your first on call shift.

HANDOVER

Handing over is important for the continuity of care. The handover process between the day and night teams is critical in ensuring the sickest patients receive the required attention overnight, when the staff strength is lower compared to the day time. Every department in each Trust has its handover process which includes the venue, time and system used. The system used may require passwords; ensure you have those passwords and if they are stored on specific drives, check to ascertain that you have been granted the required level of access.

If you take on additional locum shifts within your Trust, in a different department, be sure to obtain this information as different departments operate differently. Keep a personal record of information handed over as well as those you hand over. In situations where care provided is challenged, one of the key things assessed is the continuity of care provided. For example, when did the patient start to show signs of deterioration, what interventions were put in place and how was the patient followed up to ensure the interventions led to improvement. Invariably, such patients will need to be monitored closely.

If you were a member of the day team, this means ensuring you hand over the patient for review overnight. If you are a member of the night team, there should be evidence that you received the information to review the patient. If an attempt is made to cast blame, those records can serve as a source of vindication.

ON CALL

'Being on call' means that you are a member of the admitting team. This also means you will receive referrals from the

Accident and Emergency (A and E) department and you may also receive referrals from General Practitioners (phone calls or electronic referrals). The on call team will also be responsible for managing patients who become critically unwell when the day shift is over.

It is useful to know the escalation plan when you are on call – who do you report to and how do you communicate with that person when you are on call. Typically, it is hierarchical; the F1 doctor to F2 or SHO, SHO to Registrar, Registrar to Consultant. This is not always the case, so ensure you have clarity on who you report to. Document any escalations, include the time the call was made and to whom it was made. Also document the action plan discussed.

In my own case, I was very unprepared for my first on call shift which also happened to be a night shift. My consultant instructed me to call him if I had any doubt. I was an SHO and there was no Registrar support at night. I called the consultant for every patient and was not even prepared with information like lab test results and imaging reports.

As a result, I got terrible feedback. However, I learnt quickly and subsequently called overnight only for patients who might need surgery. More so, I had all the facts the consultant needed for decision making.

Calling your senior to discuss patients is a skill. It is tested in many interviews and course settings. If it is necessary to make a call to a senior, get feedback on what you did well and aspects you can do better.

DOCUMENTATION

In the practice of Medicine, there is a popular adage which says, "If it is not documented, it did not happen." Any patient review, interaction with their relatives, changes in management plans, etc., should be documented.

For documentation purposes, the title of the review should be stated. For example, in consultant ward round, state the name of the consultant reviewing the patient. If you are documenting the review by a senior colleague, at the end, state your full name and role. You may receive a stamp which has your GMC number; this can be used in addition to your name and role.

On night shift reviews, state the reason you are reviewing the patient. That is, were you told to see the patient by the nursing staff, a junior colleague or was the patient handed over for review. This assists the day team to quickly understand the challenges faced overnight and how they were addressed.

RADIOLOGY

Requesting radiological investigations often require that you undergo training. Thereafter, access will be granted to request and view investigations. Your position or hierarchy determines the type of investigations that can be requested. While some investigations require that a registrar reviews the patient first, some others require a consultant.

Before requesting investigations, review the previous imaging of the patient and how recent investigations were conducted. Some investigations require speaking with the radiographer or radiologist for approval. Prior to making the phone call, be clear on the clinical history of the patient and how the investigation will change the course of clinical management. Even though your authority to request the investigation may be challenged, remember that all teams are working for the best outcome of the patient.

However, the clinical team have the upper hand of having reviewed the patient; so if an investigation you deem necessary is refused by the radiology team, escalate to a more senior member of your team and document all discussions.

ACCESS TO GP RECORDS

Access to GP records of a patient is not automatically granted. Patients who are referred from the GP may come with a printed record, which contains medical history of previous ailments and current repeat medications. For patients who will be admitted to the hospital, it is imperative that they receive their regular medications while on admission.

If a patient is unable to provide information about her regular medications, request permission from that patient to access the GP's records and obtain the information. In most Trusts, the pharmacy team will cross check the prescription chart to ensure the patient is only receiving currently prescribed medications.

Again, access to GP records is typically not automatic. Make enquiries on how to obtain access and ensure you have it by your first time on call.

DRUG PRESCRIPTIONS

Prescribing may be electronic or handwritten. The principles remain the same. Choose the drug, route of administration, the duration of administration and review date. If there are any changes to regular medications, it should be included in the discharge summary sent to the GP. Treatment guidelines, particularly for antibiotic use, are in place in most Trusts.

It is helpful to be familiar with how to access them. Antibiotic stewardship is the responsibility of every clinician. Pharmacists and microbiologists will regularly challenge whatever they consider as inappropriate use. When in doubt, ask.

In summary, in hospital settings in the UK, you are not expected to prescribe antibiotics randomly. Rather, follow predetermined guidelines and ask for support from the microbiology team if you have any challenges.

For allergies, documentation is done on the drug chart by the admitting clinician. It is also the responsibility of every clinician, who prescribes medications, to ensure that a patient is not allergic to the medication being prescribed. For patients you review, make sure no drug prescribed, whether by you or otherwise, can do them harm.

Therefore, review the drug chart and check that everything is appropriate, so far as you have reviewed that patient. For example, check that the dosage of medications a patient with renal impairment is receiving is appropriate for them.

INTERACTION WITH OTHER
TEAM MEMBERS

The UK is well ahead when it comes to recognising the value of every team member. For example, a surgeon may perform a successful hip replacement but the timing of discharge is dependent on the physiotherapist and occupational therapist.

When you join a new team, find out the work process. Are there specialist nurses? What is your role in relation to theirs? What support is available to you? For example, the tissue viability nurses will look after pressure sores in some Trusts. In other Trusts, pain team nurses will review pain and optimise pain control, palliative team for palliative care, etc. Learning about these support systems will happen as you get familiar with the system. Awareness of the support systems is the first step; the next step is understanding when to deploy them to your advantage.

COMMUNICATING WITH PATIENTS
AND THEIR RELATIVES

The content of this section may seem basic but as

with life, the simplest things can make all the difference. When approaching a patient, greet first before explaining why you are there to see him/her. If the patient had a long wait to see you, offer an apology and an explanation.

Assuming the patient has a companion, ask about the relationship that exists between them and whether the patient is comfortable having the companion present for the clinical review. The companion may be uncomfortable with being present for the examination of the patient, so check again before clinical examination.

When a diagnosis is reached, explain it to the patient. For cancer diagnosis, the discussion is usually reserved for senior members of the team. You may intimate the patient that you are concerned about the symptoms and signs, but cannot make a conclusive diagnosis.

Decisions about palliation, 'Do Not Resuscitate' orders and ceiling of care are usually made with the consultant. However, discussion of this decision with relatives can be left to any member of the team. It is useful to witness this discussion before engaging in it for the first time.

It is also advised that you document every discussion, stating the subject matter, participants and witnesses of the discussion. For example, the discussion could have been with the daughter of the patient (name clearly documented) with the ward sister present.

It is also useful to document whether it was a physical discussion or over the phone. If it was held over the phone, document the phone number used as well. No matter the nature of communication, ensure you clarify that the other party understands the reason for the communication and the information that was communicated.

Undoubtedly, there will be comments about difficulty in understanding your accent. Take the comments in your stride and do not let them interfere with the good job you are doing.

DO NOT ATTEMPT CARDIOPULMONARY RESUSCITATION (DNACPR)

DNACPR or Do Not Attempt Resuscitation (DNAR) is a clinical decision that is made with the knowledge of the patient and where possible, their relatives as well. This decision can be made by a senior clinician but ideally, should be signed by a consultant for full validity. The DNAR order is not synonymous with a ceiling of care.

The DNAR simply means that if the patient has a cardiac arrest, no attempt will be made to resuscitate due to poor outcomes expected. If a patient has a DNAR in place from the community, usually signed by the GP, a hospital DNAR order will still need to be instituted.

The ceiling of care is a directive that can be instituted by the managing consultant, the palliative or the outreach team. It lays out the level of care a patient should receive. When called to review a patient, after initial assessment, review the notes to obtain critical information like the ceiling of care decided as well as the patient's DNAR status. If the clinical status is such that death is imminent, it is usually expected that a member of the team notifies the family.

CRASH CALL

A loud buzzer goes off when any health worker identifies a patient that is at risk of or has undergone cardiopulmonary arrest. Whilst there is a dedicated CRASH team, health workers within the vicinity of the CRASH call are expected to act first. The most senior person at the scene often takes the lead role and assigns task until the designated CRASH team arrives and there is a handover. Sometimes, the CRASH call is a drill using a dummy. You are expected to take the drill seriously and resuscitate the dummy.

BULLYING

Although the definition of bullying is standard, the situations in which people feel bullied are different. Since you are from a different country, you may experience situations where you are spoken to in a derogatory manner on account of your race, skin tone or even your accent. The things that make you a unique being can become objects of ridicule.

Bullying can come from any direction. Ward nurses may question your valid decisions; doctors of junior rank may ignore your instructions or bypass you to seek counsel from locally trained colleagues. Seniors may make snide remarks that undermine your authority. While some of the behaviours will be worth challenging or reporting, others can be defused without escalation.

These experiences may wear down your confidence; however, the first way to protect yourself is to understand that the prejudices you are experiencing are not personal, but represent a culture of treating IMGs as incompetent. The second way is to arm yourself with knowledge, so you blend into the system quicker and with less glitches.

It is important not to let bullies get away with their actions; however, it is more important to be mindful of what you allow into your consciousness. Pick battles carefully and do not become the person who attributes every criticism to racism. When addressing rude behaviour, report the facts without sensationalism. Choose wisely the person you report to, in order to avoid worsening the situation.

The most important tip here is to find support in the friendships you build. Other immigrants have had these experiences before you and will provide invaluable tips to navigate difficult situations. Also, the office of the Freedom to Speak Up Guardian potentially provides an opportunity to raise concerns confidentially.

The NHS as an organisation frowns heavily at discrimination and bullying for any reason. Even the prime minister has weighed in, making it clear that racism will not be tolerated from patients to NHS staff. However, the reality remains far from the ideal.

CHAPTER 4

PARENTING

The NHS is very supportive of family life. If your family expands, either via pregnancy or adoption, there are paid leave options for both parents. Refer to the policy guidelines in your Trust.

Pregnancy is a miracle. It is a physiological state and not a disease. You may have to remember this, if you become pregnant while working. For instance, you may no longer be able to go for the same period of time without food, drink or bathroom breaks. Your attention span may change, stamina may reduce, and you may experience difficulties that you did not anticipate.

On the other hand, you may be absolutely fine with no one aware that you are pregnant until it becomes visible. Whatever your situation is, know that you are not alone and there are systems in place to support you.

NOTIFYING YOUR CLINICAL LEAD

It is important to make early plans to inform your clinical lead about your pregnancy. This notification should be done in writing. Understand that the timing of the notification can affect your maternity payment. So, ensure to read the NHS Maternity Leave and Pay guide if you plan to get pregnant or are pregnant.

The line manager/clinical lead should then go through a form called 'work place assessment' with you. During this process, your daily duties and surroundings will be assessed for their suitability to your pregnancy. This assessment includes contact with infectious material, handling heavy things, sitting arrangements, etc.

ATTENDING YOUR APPOINTMENTS

Notify the rota co-ordinator and your line supervisor about your hospital appointments. They are expected to make arrangements so you can attend them without using your annual leave days.

ILL HEALTH DURING PREGNANCY

Any time taken off due to a pregnancy related illness should not be recorded as part of your sick leave. If you have difficulties such as bleeding, high blood pressure, etc., in pregnancy, it is worth informing the occupational health team, so that they can assess you and adjust your shifts if necessary.

MAT B1 FORM

This is a certificate that confirms the pregnancy to your employer and notifies them about when the baby is expected. The form, which should not be completed more than twenty weeks before you are due, is filled by your midwife or doctor. Make a copy of the completed form before handing it over to your payroll team.

Most Trusts have a standard application form used to apply for maternity leave and it may need to be submitted with the Mat B1 form. Apart from getting time off, the purpose of this application is to assess your eligibility for maternity payment. There is a maternity pay calculator online that provides a guide, so you know if you can expect to be paid and the duration of payment during your maternity leave.

Although the maternity pay is dependent on duration of service, time off is not. Every pregnant woman is entitled to 52 weeks of maternity leave - twenty-six weeks paid leave, if eligible and twenty-six weeks without pay (although you may be eligible for statutory maternity pay during that period). Your payroll department should inform you about your eligibility as the outcome of your application. You are unlikely to qualify for payment if you have worked less than a year in the NHS. Choose your return date carefully because it may not be easily changed once the maternity leave starts.

KEEPING IN TOUCH DAYS

You may discuss going to work during your maternity leave to support the team. These days are paid work days and can be discussed with your line manager. There is paper work to be completed and signed if you choose this option.

ANNUAL LEAVE

Maternity leave is exclusive of your annual leave. You are expected to take the annual leave that accrues. Plan the annual and maternity leave in a manner that allows you take what you are entitled to. It is important to note that you get paid during annual leave. For example, you may begin by taking two weeks of annual leave before your due date and then start maternity leave from your due date. That gives you the opportunity to maximise the maternity leave.

PENSION

All NHS staff are automatically enrolled in a pension scheme. This pension is deducted monthly from your salary. Depending on your years of employment with the NHS, you may be able to apply for a refund on the contributions you have made if you are eligible.

Regardless of the possibility to get a refund on the pension contributions, it is also possible to opt out of it. That way, the contribution is not deducted from the maternity pay.

SICKNESS

It can be difficult to overcome the reluctance to call in sick. There is nothing wrong with admitting you are unwell and will be unable to cope with work. This is particularly important, especially if the sickness is infectious. You may self-certify an illness for a limited time; check local guidelines with your employer. If the sickness persists, a sick note from the doctor will be required.

There will be a protocol for reporting sickness and what to do when you resume work. Be aware and follow the local guidelines.

It is important to note that there is usually a maximum amount of sick days that is permissible. Beyond this point, there may be meetings about adjusting your work schedule and this may affect your pay. For people on sponsored visas, there are earning thresholds. So, if you find yourself in this situation, make sure you have assessed the implications thoroughly.

Furthermore, new employers will usually ask your previous employer how much time was taken off work due to ill health.

It requires courage to not go to work because of ill health. I have heard consultants berate people for taking sick leave while praising others for working in spite of being ill. This is unhealthy! Do not feel pressured to work when you are unwell. Errors are imminent when your health is suboptimal.

Unfortunately, being unwell is not an acceptable defence if anything that leads to patient harm occurs. It is unwise to compromise your health for the sake of service. On the other hand, it can feel like you are letting your team down. Learn to put your health first!

CHAPTER 5

APPRAISALS

In this chapter, I will discuss appraisals – how to get involved in teaching, quality improvement projects and making the most of a single activity. There will also be a brief discussion about building portfolios.

You may likely hear locally trained doctors talk about their portfolios. This is essentially your CV but a bit more elaborate. For training jobs, which we will discuss in the next chapter, applicants may need to present portfolios that showcase their achievements for review by interviewers. Regardless of whether you opt to go into a training programme or not, it is important to build your portfolio and model it around what is expected of trainees in your specialty.

The first time you may likely compile evidence will be for the GMC mandated annual appraisal. An assumption that often gets IMGs into difficult situations is the expectation that all required information will be provided. There are many Trusts where this is not the case. Outlined below is the information you need to make the most of your appraisal. First, you should be assigned an appraiser within your Trust.

This should happen automatically with a notification e-mail about your appraiser. You may also get a provisional appraisal date at this time. You should be given login details to the web application that your Trust uses for appraisals; log in and see what it looks like. Usually, the appraisal takes place some months into your role. The appraisal meeting is not automatic; so you will need to arrange a convenient time and place with your appraiser.

It is important to look at the appraisal web application well ahead of time, to enable a good understanding of expected questions and provide evidence, if necessary. Some key sections are highlighted below.

CONTINUING PROFESSIONAL DEVELOPMENT (CPD)

Keeping an accurate record of CPD points can be tricky. Formal courses will typically state the number of points earned. However, studying and attending clinical meetings also attract points. It is helpful to read and familiarize yourself with the GMC's guidance for CPD (see additional resources for link).

REVIEW OF COMPLAINTS AND COMPLIMENTS

Complaints tend to be more readily given than compliments. If a complaint is made about you, it may seem harsh or painful especially when you are new and putting in your best. Learn the important lesson from the event and do not dwell on it beyond the learning. If you receive a written complaint, you are expected to discuss it with your appraiser. Ensure that you can demonstrate what you learnt from the situation.

Compliments, which can be scarce, are also tricky to obtain for junior doctors or doctors in emergency settings. You may consider asking someone who paid you a compliment if they would not mind putting it in writing.

PERSONAL DEVELOPMENT PLAN PROPOSALS

This outlines the goals you want to work towards before your next appraisal. It is helpful to have three goals with varying levels of difficulty – one fairly easy to achieve goal, an intermediate goal and a difficult goal. At your next appraisal, you will need to ascertain whether or not you achieved these goals; so it is helpful to be realistic. You will need your employer's support to achieve your documented goals. For example, if you have a professional examination as a goal, you are more likely to get study leave approved.

TEACHING

Teaching is a very important aspect of practice in the UK and the GMC wants evidence that you are participating in it. A lot of teaching in medical practice happens informally but some are formal. It is very likely that the Trust already has formal teaching programmes for medical students or foundation doctors.

Find out who is in charge and how you can participate. Do not give up if you face any difficulty. Try with someone different until you are able to get the opportunity you need.

Collecting evidence of teaching is just as important as the teaching itself. Feedback forms can easily be found online and adapted if you are doing the teaching. For example, if you teach medical students in a bedside session, you can give them feedback forms to complete for you.

If you have attended a teaching session, be sure to sign attendance. Evidence of attending teaching can be used for your appraisal in the CPD section.

If there is no formal teaching programme in your Trust or department, you can organise one. This can be used as evidence for leadership. Speak with a consultant to get support to implement the teaching programme. It is also useful to speak with potential recipients of the teaching to ensure there is adequate interest. In summary, one way or another, engage in teaching and collect evidence of your teaching activities.

QUALITY IMPROVEMENT

This includes audits and quality improvement projects. Another aspect of this is the use of Datix system. The subsequent sections will elaborate on how to engage in each of these optimally.

DATIX INCIDENT REPORTING SYSTEM

This is a web-based application that allows individuals report events that caused or had the potential to cause harm. Ideally, it should be used objectively and lead to learning. It still fulfils ideal objectives but is also used vindictively. If you are named in a Datix, you may or may not be informed.

If you are informed, you will be told what is expected of you. It usually entails explaining your involvement in the reported event.

AUDIT

Clinical audits assess performance against accepted standards. They are useful for improving the quality of care provided to patients. A completed audit cycle implies that following an audit, a deficiency was found, a quality improvement (QI) project was designed and executed, and a second audit was carried out to assess the effectiveness of the QI project in correcting the deficit found from the first audit.

Choosing an audit for the first time requires skill. It is important to select a topic that is relevant to the team and interesting to you. A common mistake is picking a topic that is of interest to you and expecting it to be interesting to everyone. To avoid this mistake, speak with teammates who deal with the unit's data as well as the consultants, to find out areas they are interested in auditing that align with your interests.

There are national audits in various specialty areas where you can see firsthand an area in which your hospital is underperforming. This affords you the opportunity to go straight to designing a QI project to improve performance. Once you have implemented the changes in your project, from the data submitted, you can assess how the project impacted the quality of patient care.

Quality improvement is designed to improved patient care; however, participating in projects provides opportunities to develop useful career skills like leadership and team building. Another skill that can be learnt is oral and poster presentation skills. Prior to an audit, it is helpful to present an audit proposal to the team. If this opportunity is missed, then the QI project should be presented. This sensitizes the team about the changes they can expect.

Following the implementation of the QI project, there should be an audit of performance. This serves as a project report and should be presented to the team. Annual conferences of trainee groups and specialties take place in the UK with calls for oral and poster presentations. Make efforts to submit your work and have it presented at a regional meeting.

This way, a single project affords opportunities to showcase leadership and presentation skills as well as engagement in QI activities.

ACHIEVEMENTS AND CHALLENGES

It is easy to undervalue your achievements and imagine you have nothing to document in this section. If you have organised any audit, QI project or teaching, it should be included here. To make the most of your time, volunteer whenever your consultants need someone to perform an audit or represent the team. Also volunteer to be the local junior lead for national and international projects such as the Global Surg data collaborative.

It may be difficult to be open about challenges you have faced without making it seem like a complaint. The key here is to highlight what made the situation difficult without much detail about the difficulty.

SIGNIFICANT EVENTS

These are unexpected or unintended events which led to or had the potential to lead to harm. They are different from complaints. If you are named in any significant event, you will receive written correspondence to that effect and it is mandatory to disclose this during your appraisal. If you fail to include it, your appraisal team who would have been notified will bring it to the attention of your appraiser.

COLLEAGUE AND PATIENT FEEDBACK

The web-based appraisal application can be used to collect feedback from colleagues. As a rule of thumb, ask more people than you need for feedback, so as to get the required number in good time. As important as it is to get honest feedback, it serves no purpose to ask people you do not get along with. All documentation can and will be used against you, if you are involved in any case.

360-degree (multi-source) feedback is needed once per revalidation cycle, which is typically once in five years. It collates feedback from colleagues across health disciplines. Apart from the fact that it is decent to be nice and respectful to everyone, it makes it easier to request help with completing your multi-source feedback.

Patient feedback is a bit more challenging to collect as you have to explain its purpose and do not want to create the impression of being nice because you want positive feedback. To resolve this, ask for help from the nursing staff or ward clerks. They can help you discuss the form and its purpose with patients. That way, the form is only handed to you when the patient completes it and you are not directly involved.

CHAPTER 6

PLANNING FOR THE FUTURE

Once you have settled into your first job, it is useful to start thinking about the future. Career trajectories are often disrupted by relocation; thus, there is a need to adjust expectations accordingly. Career planning will depend on the level of training and specialisation.

It is important to understand the system to reduce the chances of being disappointed. The system rewards employers for prioritising the training of trainees. Doctors in non-training positions are essentially service providers and no incentive exists to train them. Carla Harris delivered an amazing TED talk titled, "How to find the person who can help you get ahead at work".

This is an insightful video to watch for IMGs, because you will invariably need someone to support you when renewing your contract or choosing people to work with on projects. For doctors in skill-based jobs like surgery, it can also be useful to have people who want the best outcomes for you. They will give you the opportunities to acquire skills.

Training programmes for IMGs can seem very daunting to achieve, particularly, when all the requirements are unknown. Arming yourself with all the necessary information, as well as finding a senior who knows the system to guide you, will put you in the best position to succeed.

MEDICAL CV IN THE UK

Medical CV in the UK is structured such that each section begins on a new page. Sections include, but are not limited to, education, teaching, publications, leadership and management. Traditionally, repetition is frowned upon in CVs. However, for medical CV, achievements that cut across different sections can be repeated. Chronological arrangement within the sections is not strictly necessary. The most important achievements can be highlighted at the top of the page. It is helpful to see a colleague's CV for guidance.

CHOOSING A SPECIALTY

Medical school exposes students to various specialties and the foundation years reveal life as it is in a given specialty. It can be difficult to choose a specialty. Before you make a decision, consider your values, how much time you want to devote to family, extracurricular activities, etc.

People spend three to four decades working after specialisation; so it is important to choose an aspect you enjoy and not base your choice on a specialty being easy to get into. Competition ratios from the previous year are usually available. They provide guidance to applicants, which may be reviewed in one of two ways. If the competition is steep, prepare adequately so you stand out or find a less competitive specialty.

Always remember that specialty training is not binding. There's always the opportunity to opt out and do what you enjoy, either by retraining in a different specialty or changing your career track.

SPECIALTY TRAINING

IMGs who have completed foundation training within or outside the UK are eligible to apply for specialty or GP training. Depending on the level of experience, the applicant may apply for Core, Run Through or Specialty Training. Core Training starts at CT1 and specialty training from ST3 or ST4, depending on the specialty.

Run Through post means that trainees start at CT1 and do not have to reapply at ST3, but continue their training after which they obtain a Certificate of Completion of Training (CCT). Uncoupled programmes mean that following completion of Core Training, if you aspire to Specialty Training, then, you will need to go through another round of Specialty application.

Popular belief for IMGs is that obtaining a National Training Number (NTN) is too difficult. I disagree with this notion! If you understand the system and what is expected, you will attain your dreams. Notwithstanding, some dreams will be more difficult to achieve than others.

The key question is, how badly do you want it? There will be people who believe certain specialties are reserved for UK trainees and this may steer you towards specialties that seem easier to attain training into. It is your life and you owe it to yourself to at least try for what you want.

ANNUAL REVIEW OF COMPETENCY PROGRESSION (ARCP)

In the previous chapter, we examined the annual appraisal process where competencies and their progression are assessed for doctors not in training jobs. The ARCP is the equivalent system for doctors in training. The expected achievements for the year are clearly laid out and candidates have meetings with their supervisors before the final meeting outcome.

Trainees, who are struggling to meet the required expectations, will be supported in deficiency areas.

ELIGIBILITY EXAMINATIONS

Multi-Specialty Recruitment Assessment

Multi-Specialty Recruitment Assessment (MSRA) is a computer-based assessment used for entry into postgraduate medical training for the following specialties: General Practice, Psychiatry (Core and Child and Adolescent Mental Health Services), Radiology, Ophthalmology, Obstetrics and Gynaecology, Community and Sexual Reproductive Health, and Neurosurgery.

The MSRA examination result is valid for one recruitment cycle. That is, one year. Each of the specialties uses the score in different ways for their national recruitment process. Therefore, it is advisable to visit the national recruitment site, for your specialty of choice, to understand expectations.

College Membership Examination

Examples of college examination include Membership of the Royal College of Surgeons (MRCS), Membership of the Royal College of Physicians (MRCP), etc. These examinations are typically not required for core training in any of the specialties, but can serve as bonus points showing commitment to the specialty. They are usually in parts and must be passed in order to commence specialty training or progress to specialty level for run through programmes. Most of the examinations have a maximum number of attempts. It is useful to be aware of this before attempting them.

As IMGs, membership examination and indeed all examinations pose a new challenge. Since you are being tested in a system that differs from that in which you were trained, it is advisable to attend a course, particularly for those with Objective Structured Clinical Examinations (OSCE). Each College publishes their examination information, so that is a useful place to start.

Pay attention to information like the number of times the examination is given in a year and how the timing relates to application timelines. This will give you adequate time to pass the examination before applications open.

Fellowship Examination

In some Royal colleges, a fellowship examination may qualify you for fellowship in the college while in other colleges, members need to be nominated to fellowship status. In the latter group, fellowship status is not a mark of completion of training; rather, it is an award to distinguish a member for excellent service rendered.

For example, the Royal Colleges of Surgery and Ophthalmology award Fellowships for completion of examinations. That is, fellowship by examination. For medical specialties, there are no fellowship examinations; the Specialty Certificate Examination is used instead. Fellows are nominated and awarded the prestigious accolade, fellowship by award.

For GP Specialty Training (GPST), to attain CCT you need to pass the MRCGP examination which is in two-parts – Applied Knowledge Test (AKT) and Clinical Skills Assessment. Research your specialty of interest to understand what obtains.

Some colleges accept qualifications from overseas training programmes and these are published on the GMC website. The GMC will also accept a letter from a Royal College for the purpose of recognising overseas qualifications.

PREPARING FOR INTERVIEWS

The interview process for each specialty is different. It is highly recommended that you obtain preparatory materials and attend courses where available. It is also important to practice with people who will attend the interview as well.

Some Trusts organise mock interviews for employees who are attending interviews. In the absence of an existing system, this can be organised by anyone, with support from consultants who are familiar with the selection process. For IMGs who have no experience of National selection, the Mock is very valuable.

GMC SPECIALTY REGISTER

The GMC specialty register is a list of doctors who meet the eligibility criteria to take up fixed term, honorary or substantive consultant posts in a UK health service. Locum consultants are not required to be listed on the specialist register.

Although a doctor may practice in a specialty not shown on their specialist register entry, they must be listed on the specialist register to practice as consultants in any UK health service.

Recognised routes to apply to be on the Speciality register include CCT or CESR CP, which is obtained after training in GMC approved training posts.

You can also obtain Certificate of Eligibility for Specialist Register (CESR) or Certificate of Eligibility for GP registration (CEGPR).

CERTIFICATE OF ELIGIBILITY FOR SPECIALIST REGISTER – COMBINED PROGRAMME (CESR CP) VS CESR

Trainees who have had their trainings in GMC approved training posts, that is Foundation, Core and Speciality training will receive a CCT at the end of their training, regardless of whether it was a run through training or not.

Trainees who completed part of their training in non-GMC approved posts such as overseas qualified doctors, who enter specialty training, will obtain a CESR CP. Doctors who are unable to get into training programmes are allowed to submit evidence, for consideration to be listed on the specialty register.

The CESR route requires a lot of commitment. It can be quite daunting when no support is given to attain the same goals that trainees are heavily supported to achieve. Generally, it is considered more difficult; however, it is achievable with commitment and patience.

SAS DOCTORS

Specialty and Associate Specialist (SAS) Doctors are a diverse group of doctors, with varying levels of skill and expertise, who contribute a significant amount to the specialty work force. Efforts are ongoing to standardise and support them as a group.

This option is suited to people who neither intend to become consultants nor go through training programmes.

NON-HOSPITAL ROLES

Various opportunities exist outside traditional clinical roles for medically qualified graduates. These include roles in pharmaceutical companies, medical device companies, functional assessors, consulting jobs, etc.

Think about your values, what you want to accomplish in life, how you like to spend your time and decide the best route for you to achieve your dreams. There will be people who believe certain specialties are reserved for UK trainees and they may steer you towards specialties that seem easier to access for training. It is your life and you owe it to yourself to at least try for what you want.

CHAPTER 7

MY EXPERIENCE

When I moved to the United Kingdom, I was neither black nor an ethnic minority. Rather, I was a confident, pregnant, married woman who temporarily left her family in pursuit of her career aspirations. I was a high achiever!

I had just completed my second year of training and was one of nine successful applicants selected out of nearly a hundred, for Plastic Surgery Residency. I was also one of a thousand applicants selected out of four thousand, for the Tony Elumelu Foundation Entrepreneurship Grant. I was running a thriving healthcare recruitment business as well as a successful Non-Governmental Organisation (NGO) in youth empowerment. No doubt, I was a very confident woman.

In my first job, I suffered emotional abuse from colleagues, which goes well beyond the scope of this book to describe. However, I will give examples. The staff services team were short staffed, so I was bullied into doing three extra night shifts. Meanwhile, they had no intention to pay me for these extra shifts. A month later, when I again found myself in an unfair situation, I raised the issue of an emerging pattern of bullying. My educational supervisor was engaged and thankfully, supported me even when the clinical lead did not. I got paid and that was a small victory.

I had colleagues who compiled cases against me that were outright lies. They sent an e-mail to the consultant stating that I was not competent with patient care. I was fortunate because my good work exonerated me.

When the Human Resource Officer learnt that I was pregnant, she wrote to the home office stating that I had taken advantage of the NHS and would have to pay for the care I received as a pregnant woman. I had to furnish evidence that I had paid for the international health surcharge before the issue was cleared.

Irrespective of these bad experiences, at the same hospital, I had good experiences. One of the consultants from the panel that interviewed me was impressed with my achievements prior to joining the Trust. He asked about my career aspirations and directed me to see two other consultants, who were instrumental in telling me how the system was structured and how to build my portfolio. One of them gave me the opportunity to get involved with my first audit, which led to a poster presentation at a regional meeting as well as a publication.

A different consultant, with whom I worked regularly, was my first appraiser. I had asked for help with my portfolio which was not forthcoming. I did my best but it was not good enough. Notwithstanding, he was not put off. Instead, he spent the appraisal meeting telling me how to go about things. He shared invaluable knowledge that helped me to quickly develop professionally; some are documented in this book.

I proceeded to participate in my first QI project, which led to an oral presentation at a regional meeting as well as training in QI processes. One of the registrars advised me on how to get ahead, put myself forward and improve the confidence my bosses had in me.

It is needless to say that by the time I left my first job, although I had learnt a lot, I was no longer the confident woman that arrived in the UK. I became the label – migrant doctor. A label which is not itself offensive but carries lower expectations of knowledge.

When I arrived at my second job, I resumed with an on-call shift. I did not have access to all the systems used and by some process glitch, I had not received the manual that explained the operation process in the unit. I spent the first week completely disoriented and committing all kinds of unwitting blunders. The consultant on call was put off and breathing down my neck, making it even more difficult for me to feel settled.

It took some time and support from friends and family before I eventually regained my confidence. My renewed confidence gave me the courage to apply to be a staff governor for my Foundation Trust. I secured enough votes to be offered the position when the winner left the Trust. By the time I was leaving this job, I got compliments about my confidence and how much I had changed since joining.

Thinking about my experiences, I knew that I did not want others to go through the hardships I endured. I guided friends and helped them navigate the system with the knowledge I acquired. It was delightful to see them thrive socially and in their careers.

When I think about my early days in the system, I see clearly the errors I made and how they influenced the way I was treated by others. The desire I have, is for no one to experience the demoralisation that comes from lack of knowledge of simple things when getting to know a new system.

This book has been written to direct you to ask the right questions. I hope everyone who reads it feels better equipped to thrive in a medical career in the UK.

ADDITIONAL RESOURCES

1. General Medical Council website 2020 CPD Guidance Available from: https://www.gmc-uk.org/education/standards-guidance-and-curricula/guidance/continuing-professional-development

2. Gov.UK 2020 Driving licence https://www.gov.uk/driving-nongb-licence/y/a-resident-of-great-britain/full-car-and-motorcycle/any-other-country7

3. UK Foundation Programme Office 2020 Available from: ttps://www.google.com/url?sa=t&source=web&rct=j&url=https://www.foundationprogramme.nhs.uk/wp-content/uploads/sites/2/2019/11/UKFP-2020-Eligibility-Applicant-

4. Guidance 0.pdf&ved=2ahUKEwjrlrOpyeboAhUExoUKHV61AE4QFjAAegQIBBAC&usg=AOvVaw0bog99BkEWQFGewGqZnEir

5. Health Education England 2020 Available from: https://www.google.com/url?sa=t&source=web&rct

6. =j&url=https://heeoe.hee.nhs.uk/sites/default/files/msra_test_blueprint_information_nov_2019.pdf&ved=2ahUKEwiyzMbm4-foAhWoVBUIHXKuA5gQFjABegQIBBAI&usg=AOvVaw2UvR4rjIETc2vF75MvxesL

7. Health Education England 2020 GP Recruitment Available from: https://gprecruitment.hee.nhs.uk/recruitment/

8. Royal College of Obstetricians and Gynaecologists 2020 Membership Categories Available from://www.rcog.org.uk/en/about-us/membership/membership-categories/#fellows

9. Royal College of Ophthalmology 2020 Membership categories Available from: https://www.rcophth.ac.uk/about/membership-overview/membership-categories/

10. Royal College of Physicians 2020 Fellowship Available from: https://www.rcplondon.ac.uk/fellowship

11. Health Education England 2020 Specialty Training Available from: https://specialtytraining.hee.nhs.uk/ARCP

12. Royal College of General Practitioners 2020 GP Training Available from: https://www.rcgp.org.uk/training-exams/discover-general-practice/qualifying-as-a-gp-in-the-nhs/certificate-of-eligibility-for-gp-registration-combined-programme-route-cegpr-cp.aspx

13. Oriel2020 Login page Available from: https://www.oriel.nhs.uk/Web/Account/LandingPage

ABOUT THE AUTHOR

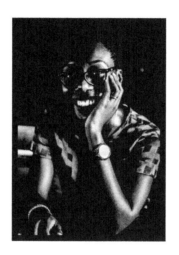

IBIFUNKE PEGBA-OTEMOLU studied Medicine at Kwame Nkrumah University of Science and Technology, Ghana. Thereafter, she moved back to Nigeria to practice. After a couple of years, she pursued and earned a Masters' degree in International Health Management from the Imperial College Business School, London. She worked as an Intern with Philips Research in Eindhoven, Netherlands, before returning to Nigeria.

She was accepted into the Plastic Surgery Residency Programme at the National Orthopaedic Hospital, Igbobi, Lagos. After a while, she relocated to the UK where she started out as a Senior House Officer in Orthopaedics and Trauma. Subsequently, she worked as a Trust Grade Core Trainee in General Surgery at the Oxford University Hospitals NHS Foundation Trust, where she also served as a Staff Governor in the Foundation Trust's Council of Governors. She works as a specialty doctor in Northern Lincolnshire UK, where she is pursuing her aspiration to train as an Oncoplastic Breast Surgeon. She aims to build a network of breast centres in sub-Saharan Africa.

She supports medics to achieve their career aspirations through Eldorado Medic Jobs. She is also committed to youth empowerment through Ebi School Leavers' Initiative, which provides free financial literacy training and vocational skills acquisition for underprivileged youths.

Printed in Great Britain
by Amazon

78303254R00062